LOW CARB DIET

28 Days To Rapid Weight Loss, Irresistable Energy And Improve Your Lifestyle

Author: Martha Lily

Amy Simons

Editor: Healthy Eating Center

accurate, up-to-date and reliable, complete information. No warranties of any kind are expressed or implied. Readers acknowledge that the author is not engaging in the rendering of legal, financial, medical or professional advice.

By reading this document, the reader agrees that under no circumstances are we responsible for any losses, direct or indirect, which are incurred as a result of the use of information contained in this document, including, but not limited to, —errors, omissions, or inaccuracies.

Table of Contents

Introduction..1

Chapter 1: Understanding The Low Carb Diet..4

What Is A Low Carb Diet?..5

A brief history of Low-Carb Diet.............................. 6

The science behind a Low Carb Diet?....................... 8

Chapter 2: Living Healthier With Low-Carb Diet..13

Healthy benefits of Low Carb Diet...........................13

How to Start Your Low-Carb Diet............................ 15

Tips For Success Of Low Carb Diet.......................... 17

Mistakes To Avoid While On A Low Carb Diet........ 18

Chapter 3: Foods On The Low Carb Diet........... 19

Foods to consume..19

Foods to avoid.. 21

*Chapter 4: 28 Days Low-Carb Diet Meal Plan*23

Week 1 Shopping List...23

Week 1 Meal Plan..25

Week 2 Shopping List.. 33

Week 2 Meal Plan..34

Week 3 Shopping List.. 43

Week 3 Meal Plan..45

Week 4 Shopping List.. 53

Week 4 Meal Plan..55

Chapter 5: Delicious Breakfasts..........................63

1. Creamy Coconut Porridge.............................64

2. Scrambled Egg..66

3. Coconut Pancakes.....................................68

4. Devilled Eggs...70

5. Healthy Salad Sandwich...............................72

6. Warm Egg Muffins.....................................74

7. Banana Waffles..76

8. Eggplant Hash With Eggs.............................78

Chapter 6: Appetizing Lunches.........................80

9. Blue Cheese Beef Tenderloin.........................81

10. Juicy Oxtail with Gravy..............................83

11. Cedar Planked Salmon...............................85

12. Marinated Shrimp.....................................87

13. Portobello Mushroom Burger.......................89

14. Scrambled Tofu.......................................91

15. Broiled Cheesy Tilapia Parmesan...................93

16. Shrimp Etouffé..95

Chapter 7: Mouth- Watering Dinners.................97

17. Vegetable Sandwich Spread.........................98

18. Zoodles Omelet......................................100

19. Chicken Curry Salad.................................102

20. Garlic Chicken..104

21. Simple BBQ Ribs..106

22. Mushroom Pork Chops..........................108

23. Cheesy Pork Chops................................110

24. Slightly Tangy Baked Soy Lemon Chops..........112

Chapter 8: Fulfilling Snacks.............. 114

25. Tender Crisp Broccoli............................115

26. Reddy Okra And Tomatoes.................. 117

27. Roasted Garlic Cauliflower..................119

28. Sesame Green Beans............................ 121

29. Gently Fried Swiss Chard..................... 123

30. Baked Eggplant Tomato........................ 125

31. Mushroom Sauté.................................... 127

32. Prosciutto Wrapped Asparagus........... 129

Chapter 9: Amazing Deserts..................131

33. Chocolate Truffles................................. 132

34. Flowerlike Rosettes...............................134

35. Creamy Cheese Tarts.............................136

36. Faux Chocolate Mousse.........................138

37. Sticky Ganache....................................... 140

38. Crunchy Pudding Cookies..................... 142

39. Fantastic Meringues..............................144

40. Raw Candy... 146

Conclusion..148

Introduction

At first, congratulate you and thank you for buying this book and may you find it useful!

Have you ever tried too many different diets for your health? Do you want to lose your weight fast? Do you want to have better skin, better mood, and better sleep? Do you want to be more active, be full of energy, lower your blood pressure? Keep reading...

By following this amazing book, you will get all the good result of above questions. You will be more healthier, more slimmer, more stronger, more beautiful, more handsome, have better mood, better skin, better sleep, etc. just by following this low carb diet book! You will lose your excess weight and no need to be in starvation mode, meantime you can still have your favorite foods.

Low Carb Diet emphasizes that people should eat foods with low carb, high fat and proper protein. It is also called LCHF Diet. Now it is very popular around the world. As it has too many good benefits for us, not only it can help to lose weight, but also it will have many other health benefits. That's the reason why so many people follow this low carb diet. I think it will be your ideal diet considering your overall health!

So what will you find in this book?

1. Basics of low carb diet, it's history, the science behind of it

2. The benefits of low carb diet

3. Tips of successful low carb diet

4. Mistakes must be avoid

5. Foods should eat/ shouldn't eat

6. A healthy and scientific 28-day meal plan guides you a perfect low carb diet journey

7. 40 delicious and easy low carb recipes support your lifelong low carb diet advendure

8. More and more...

In total, throughout this book, you will be introduced to the most shared and basic concepts of Low-Carb Diet, followed by a healthy meal plan, as well as 40 easy to make and delicious recipes to help you kick start your diet regime! For more information, please go on reading the rest of this book, you will get what you want!

God Bless!

Martha Lily

Chapter 1: Understanding The Low Carb Diet

What Is A Low Carb Diet?

Low Carb Diet emphasizes that people should eat foods with low carb, high fat and proper protein. It is also called LCHF Diet. Now it is very popular around the world. As it has too many good benefits for us, not only it can help to lose weight, but also it will have many other health benefits, such as lower blood pressure, have better sleep, have more energy everyday, etc. That's why so many people follow this healthy diet nowadays.

In recent years, the concept of Low Carb dieting has branched into various kinds of dieting regimes such as Paleo, Ketogenic and even Atkins. They are similar, but have some differences. The primary focus of this book will be to introduce you to the fundamentals of Low-Carb dieting. Here let's come to the history of Low Carb Diet.

A brief history of Low-Carb Diet

While most people think the concept of Low-Carb diet started with the revelation of Dr. Atkins. They would be wrong. As the idea of Low-Carb diet started with the study of a London-based Undertaker from approximately 140 years ago.

The Undertaker in question was named Mr. Banting. In 1862, he was 66 years old, weighing 202 pounds, with a height of 5'5".

The problem with Banting was extreme obesity. So much that he wasn't able to see the laces of his shoes. His obesity was so severe that he began experiencing hearing problems, because fat was starting to cover his ear lobes.

He thought he was becoming deaf, and went to a throat and nose surgeon named Dr. William Harvey, who immediately detected the issue.

His prescription didn't include any medicine. Instead, it completely restricted him to a particular type of diet, which excluded sugar, starch, potatoes, and even beer!

He was permitted to consume fish, meat, wine, and vegetables, with the occasional toast.

To be exact, his regiment included each of his meals consist of:

- Six ounces of meat (poultry, fish, venison, beef, etc.).
- Any fruit pudding.
- Vegetables, except potatoes.
- His dinner, a glass of claret.
- He was allowed tea, no sugar.

Needless to say, the diet did wonders for him, and his hearing difficulties disappeared.

This inspired the doctor to carry out research and write a book based on "Low-Carb" diet, which conceived the concept of the diet.

After that, multiple scientists explored the low carb diet. But perhaps the biggest leap was when Dr. Atkins came out with the Atkins Diet.

The Atkins Diet became a popular method of losing weight, first established by cardiologist Robert C. Atkins, in 1972. The primary objective of this diet was to lower the carbohydrate intake, while placing a higher emphasis on fats and proteins.

Shortly after, Low-Carb diet experienced increased popularity, and people started to become more interested in trying it.

Eventually there were multiple variations of Low-carb diets; including diets with specific restrictions, such as the Ketogenic Diet, and Paleo Diet.

This book, though, will focus mainly on the ancient 'core' concept of Low-carb diet, established by Dr. William Harvey.

The science behind a Low Carb Diet?

One might think that the working mechanism behind this magical process might be very complicated and challenging to understand. However, I am inclined to tell you that is far from the truth.

While there are some intricate scientific phenomena going on in our body which leads to rapid weight loss, if explained in layman's terms, they are very easy to grasp.

To make it even simpler, I am going to break them down into different parts and tell you exactly how they are working in conjunction with weight loss.

Lower the level of insulin: We all know that Insulin is an imperative part of our body. It is essentially the primary hormone controlling the level of sugar in our blood.

However, another main function of insulin, aside from regulating the sugar levels, is to tell the body how much fat cells to store or how much it should carry.

In other words, Insulin manipulates two processes; lipogenesis, which is the production of fat, and at the same time inhibits lipolysis, which is supposed to burn fat.

Low-Carb diet helps to lower the body's insulin level. The graph below shows a perfect correlation between the two.

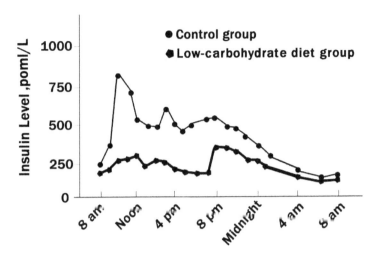

The decreased level of insulin, in turn, helps to prevent lipogenesis from taking place and increase the burning of fat through lipolysis.

A rapid reduction in water weight: When a person follows a Low-Carb diet, they tend to lose a great deal of weight during the first two weeks.

The secret behind this is primarily due to the loss of water weight.

- I have already established that a low-carb diet influences the cut down of insulin, right? When the insulin goes down, the kidneys start to shed the excess sodium from our body. Which causes the blood pressure to lower.

- This in turn, aids in preventing the body from storing carbohydrates in the form of glycogen. Once the level of carbohydrates/ glycogen in our body reduces, the water level decreases as well, since glycogen is the chemical which helps to bind water to our muscles.

A Low-Carb Diet, But High On Protein: Until now, most of the studies demonstrated that whenever a certain group takes a journey on a low carb diet, the protein intake of that group rises.

How does that help?

Protein helps to reduce appetite and increase metabolism. This helps people stay energetic throughout the day, without the need to eat constantly. This allows the body to maintain muscle mass, preventing calorie increase.

Enhanced metabolic process: While this is somewhat of a controversial claim, it is still proven that following a Low-Carb diet allows the body to increase the level of energy. This, in turn, helps the body lose more weight as well.

No more Junk food: this is perhaps the most challenging aspect of going on a Low-Carb diet. You are required to eliminate junk food.

So, sugary foods, high carbs, high lactose, artificial drinks, pastries, empty calories, processed foods are off the menu.

But please be noted the results and effectiveness of this form of diet might vary from person to person depending on their physique and metabolic stature!

Chapter 2: Living Healthier With Low-Carb Diet

Ever since the first conception of the Low-Carb diet during the 1800s, the idea of trimming down body fat by following a diet of low-carb has been mildly controversial, to put it mildly.

But that doesn't mean it has stopped people from chasing after it and trying to follow it to attain a better and healthy lifestyle!

So, now you know a bit more about the diet you plan on following. Let's explore the basic benefits you are going to experience on a Low-carb diet.

Healthy benefits of Low Carb Diet

It should be noted when beginning any new healthy regime, you should consult your physician to discuss any changes you plan on making in eating, or lifestyle. This book is meant to guide a person as they embark on low carb diet. There could be adverse effects to your health if you do not consider the illness with the change of diet. This diet is not meant to be a cure for any illness, but it could help to reduce some of the symptoms experienced.

- Could help you lose weight.
- Could reduce symptoms associated with Epilepsy.
- Could reduce acid-reflux issues.
- Could improve skin's appearance and reduce acne.
- Losing weight reduces the pressure on blood vessels and offers a freer flow of blood, which in turn could reduce the occurrence of headaches.
- Could reduce symptoms related to cardiovascular disease.
- Could reduce obesity, and improve lifestyle.
- Could reduce chances of experiencing some forms of cancer.
- Could contribute to stabilizing the levels of estrogen and progesterone.
- Could reduce the levels of triglycerides.
- Could reduce the levels of high density lipoproteins (cholesterol).

- Could reduce the levels of sugar and insulin in people affected by Diabetes, or prevent the onset of Diabetes.

Meantime, I would like you to keep an open mind when approaching the regime of Low Carb Diet because who knows what results you will attain. Like they say, don't knock it 'til you try it. This might turn out to be the life changing diet for you.

How to Start Your Low-Carb Diet

If you have decided you are going to pursue a Low-Carb diet, you might be excited to jump into the meal plans and start your diet!

But before you go hunting the shark, it is better to learn how to hunt for Tuna. What I mean by that, is you should first start by taking some small steps toward changing your eating habits before going for the whole regime.

The best way is to start cutting down carbs intake one meal at a time. Otherwise, it might be tough.

Start off by reducing your carb intake at breakfast, for one week. Then reduce the carb intake at lunch, for one week. Then reduce the carb intake at dinner for one week. Find alternative snacks with lower carbs as well.

Once you have familiarized yourself with this style of eating, you can begin the following plan.

Five things you should keep in mind when starting your journey are:

- Cut off the carbonated or sugared drink intake.
- Don't go for sweets or sugary treats.
- Avoid baked goods, pastries and biscuits.
- Avoid processed and sugary cereals.
- Avoid processed flour and processed sugars.

Tips For Success Of Low Carb Diet

- Make sure you know what kind of food you are eating, and how the different phases of Low-Carb diet works.
- Experiment and find a Low-Carb routine suitable for you.
- Keep count of your Carbohydrates.
- Be aware and sensible when choosing your portions.
- Make sure you are not starving! Eat small portions and low carbs.
- Every meal should have a protein.
- Try to opt for food made of natural fat.
- Stay away from sugar.
- Eat plenty of vegetables.
- Make sure to drink lots of water.
- Sometimes taking a vitamin can help to boost your immune system and ensure your body is not experiencing any deficiency
- Just dieting won't get you the body you desire, include some form of physical activity in your daily routine.

- Make sure to keep track of your success rate, which will further encourage you to keep moving forward

Mistakes To Avoid While On A Low Carb Diet

- Make sure when you are counting your carbs, you are going for Total Carbs instead of counting Net Carbs.
- Always make sure to not skip on vegetables.
- Don't avoid water, go for 8 cups daily at least.
- Don't completely avoid salt. A little salt never hurts.
- Don't avoid protein, each meal should have 4-6 ounces of protein.
- You are going to need to have good fat in your diet to encourage the burning of bad fat in your body.
- Failing to keep a record of your progress.

Chapter 3: Foods On The Low Carb Diet

With those details out of the way, you should have a better grasp about which foods you are actually allowed to eat and which ones you are not.

Foods to consume

- Meats such as pork, beef, chicken, lamb, and bacon.
- Fatty Fish such as trout, tilapia, salmon.
- Eggs that are rich in Omega 3.
- Low carb vegetables such as spinach, kale, asparagus.
- Full-Fat Dairy products such as butter, cream, yogurt.
- Nuts and seeds including macadamia nuts, almonds, walnuts, sunflower seeds, pumpkin seeds, and any other low fat content nuts.
- Healthy fat including extra virgin olive oil, avocado oil, and coconut oil.

Below you will find some ideas for foods and ingredients to purchase for this new lifestyle you are about to embark on.

- Fresh vegetables
- Fruits such as berries, banana, apple, pineapple etc
- Salad ingredients
- Different kinds of meats
- Sugar-free bacon
- Chicken breasts, chicken legs
- Sausages
- Steak minced or grounded
- Fish such as snapper, salmon, mussel, tuna, etc.
- Eggs
- Cheese
- Cream
- Full-Fat Yogurt
- Cream Cheese Full-Fat
- Sour Cream
- Feta
- Haloumi
- Avocado Oil
- Olive Oil
- Butter

- Coconut Oil
- Macadamia Oil
- Olives
- Canned Tomatoes
- Nuts, Seeds
- Almond Flour
- Coconut Flour
- Stevia
- Cocoa
- Unsweetened Coconut flour
- Sugar-Free Jelly
- Almond Flour Meal
- Himalayan Salt
- Herbs and Spice
- Fresh Herb
- Vinegar
- Full-Fat Mayonnaise

Foods to avoid

- Sugary drinks such as fruit juice, pop, any beverage with added sugar.
- Grains such as rye, barley, wheat.

- Oils such as corn oil, soybean oil, cottonseed oil.
- Foods with 'hydrogenated' ingredients.
- Foods with 'diet' on the label.
- High carb vegetables such as carrots and turnips. (These should be avoided during beginning phase.)
- High carb fruits such as apples, bananas, oranges. (These should be avoided during beginning phase.)
- Starches such as potatoes. (These should be avoided during beginning phase.)
- Legumes such as beans and lentils. (These should be avoided during beginning phase.)

Chapter 4: 28 Days Low-Carb Diet Meal Plan

Please note the recipes in the following Meal Plans might not be found in the recipes section provided in this book. The meal plan is prepared to give you a rough idea of how you should approach your diet. Yu can alter any of the dishes from the 40 recipes provided in the book to create your own favorite diet routine. Good luck!

Week 1 Shopping List
- Butter
- Eggs
- Coconut Flour
- Psyllium Husk Powder
- Coconut Cream
- Salt
- Coconut Milk
- Beef Tenderloin
- Teriyaki Sauce
- Red Wine
- Garlic

- Blue Cheese
- Mayonnaise
- Sour Cream
- Worcestershire Sauce
- Oxtail
- Onions
- Seasoning Salt
- Bacon Drippings
- Broth (vegetable, chicken, beef)
- Garlic Powder
- Salmon
- Black Pepper Corns
- Broccoli Florets
- Dijon Style Mustard
- Processed Cheese
- Frozen Okra
- Peppers (red, green or orange)
- Celery
- Tomatoes
- Parmesan Cheese
- Semi-sweet Chocolate Chips
- Vanilla Extract
- Condensed Milk
- Confectioner's Sugar
- Pork Chops

Week 1 Meal Plan

Day One

Total Carb Count: 22g

Breakfast:

Creamy Coconut Porridge (Calories: 322; Fat: 12.4g; Carbohydrates: 5g; Protein: 6g)

Snack

Tender Crisp Broccoli (Calories: 143; Fat: 29.28g; Carbohydrates: 7.6g; Protein: 8.6g)

Lunch

Blue Cheese Tenderloin (Calories: 280; Fat: 27g; Carbohydrates: 7g; Protein: 12g)

Snack

Reddy Okra And Tomatoes (Calories: 94; Fat: 4.7g; Carbohydrates: 1.5g; Protein: 3.8g)

Dinner

Vegetable Sandwich Spread (Calories: 42 Fat: 3.9g; Carbohydrates: 0.9g; Protein: 1g)

Dessert

Chocolate Truffles (Calories: 53; Fat: 2.5g; Carbohydrates: 7.5g; Protein: 0.9gg)

Day Two

Total Carbs Count: 30.9g

Breakfast:

Creamy Coconut Porridge (Calories: 322; Fat: 12.4g; Carbohydrates: 5g; Protein: 6g)

Snack

Sesame Green Beans (Calories: 333; Fat: 31g; Carbohydrates: 6g; Protein: 7g)

Lunch

Cedar Planked Salmon (Calories: 315; Fat: 15g; Carbohydrates: 10g; Protein: 24g)

Snack

Reddy Okra And Tomatoes (Calories: 94; Fat: 4.7g; Carbohydrates: 1.5g; Protein: 3.8g)

Dinner

Vegetable Sandwich Spread (Calories: 42; Fat: 3.9g; Carbohydrates: 0.9g; Protein: 1g)

Dessert

Chocolate Truffle (Calories: 53; Fat: 2.5g; Carbohydrates: 7.5g; Protein: 0.9gg)

<u>Day Three</u>

Total Carb Count: 46.4g

Breakfast:

Creamy Coconut Porridge (Calories: 322; Fat: 12.4g; Carbohydrates: 5g; Protein: 6g)

Snack

Tender Crisp Broccoli (Calories: 143; Fat: 29.28g; Carbohydrates: 7.6g; Protein: 8.6g)

Lunch

Marinated Shrimp (Calories: 236; Fat: 12g; Carbohydrates: 15g; Protein: 9g)

Snack

Reddy Okra And Tomatoes (Calories: 94; Fat: 4.7g; Carbohydrates: 1.5g; Protein: 3.8g)

Dinner

Portobello Mushroom Burger (Calories: 203 Fat: 14g; Carbohydrates: 9.8g; Protein: 10.3g)

Dessert

Chocolate Truffles (Calories: 53; Fat: 2.5g; Carbohydrates: 7.5g; Protein: 0.9gg)

Day Four

Total Carb Count: 34.1g

Breakfast:

Creamy Coconut Porridge (Calories: 322; Fat: 12.4g; Carbohydrates: 5g; Protein: 6g)

Snack

Baked Soy Lemon Chops (Calories: 193; Fat: 6g; Carbohydrates: 5g; Protein: 27g)

Lunch

Blue Cheese Tenderloin (Calories: 280; Fat: 27g; Carbohydrates: 7g; Protein: 12g)

Snack

Roasted Garlic Cauliflower (Calories: 118; Fat: 8.2g; Carbohydrates: 8.7g; Protein: 4.7g)

Dinner

Vegetable Sandwich Spread (Calories: 42; Fat: 3.9g; Carbohydrates: 0.9g; Protein: 1g)

Dessert

Chocolate Truffles (Calories: 53; Fat: 2.5g; Carbohydrates: 7.5g; Protein: 0.9gg)

Day Five

Total Carb Count: 32g

Breakfast:

Creamy Coconut Porridge (Calories: 322; Fat: 12.4g; Carbohydrates: 5g; Protein: 6g)

Snack

Baked Eggplant Tomato (Calories: 55; Fat: 0.38g; Carbohydrates: 9.3g; Protein: 3.3g)

Lunch

Blue Cheese Tenderloin (Calories: 280; Fat: 27g; Carbohydrates: 7g; Protein: 12g)

Snack

Gently Fried Swiss Chard (Calories: 56.2; Fat: 3.7g; Carbohydrates: 2.7g; Protein: 39g)

Dinner

Vegetable Sandwich Spread (Calories: 42 Fat: 3.9g; Carbohydrates: 0.9g; Protein: 1g)

Dessert

Chocolate Truffles (Calories: 53; Fat: 2.5g; Carbohydrates: 7.5g; Protein: 0.9gg)

Day Six

Total Carb Count: 26.2g

Breakfast:

Scrambled Eggs (Calories: 317; Fat: 26g; Carbohydrates: 1g; Protein: 19g)

Snack

Tender Crisp Broccoli (Calories: 143; Fat: 29.28g; Carbohydrates: 7.6g; Protein: 8.6g)

Lunch

Blue Cheese Tenderloin (Calories: 280; Fat: 27g; Carbohydrates: 7g; Protein: 12g)

Snack

Reddy Okra And Tomatoes (Calories: 94; Fat: 4.7g; Carbohydrates: 1.5g; Protein: 3.8g)

Dinner

Vegetable Sandwich Spread (Calories: 42; Fat: 3.9g: Carbohydrates: 0.9g; Protein: 1g)

Dessert

Flowerlike Rosettes (Calories: 561; Fat: 59g; Carbohydrates: 8.2g; Protein: 1.1g)

Day Seven

Total Carb Count: 39.3g

Breakfast:

Coconut Pancakes (Calories: 259; Fat: 15g; Carbohydrates: 6g; Protein: 4g)

Snack

Tender Crisp Broccoli (Calories: 143; Fat: 29.28g; Carbohydrates: 7.6g; Protein: 8.6g)

Lunch

Blue Cheese Tenderloin (Calories: 280; Fat: 27g; Carbohydrates: 7g; Protein: 12g)

Snack

Reddy Okra And Tomatoes (Calories: 94; Fat: 4.7g; Carbohydrates: 1.5g; Protein: 3.8g)

Dinner

Scrambled Tofu (Calories: 190 Fat: 11.5g; Carbohydrates: 9.7g; Protein: 12g)

Dessert

Chocolate Truffles (Calories: 53; Fat: 2.5g; Carbohydrates: 7.5g; Protein: 0.9gg)

Week 2 Shopping List

- Butter
- Eggs
- Coconut Flour
- Psyllium Husk Powder
- Coconut Cream
- Salt
- Coconut Milk
- Beef Tenderloin
- Teriyaki Sauce
- Red Wine
- Garlic
- Blue Cheese
- Mayonnaise
- Sour Cream
- Worcestershire Sauce
- Oxtail
- Onions
- Seasoning Salt
- Bacon Dripping
- Broth (vegetable, chicken, beef)
- Garlic Powder
- Salmon
- Black Pepper Corns
- Broccoli Florets

- Dijon Style Mustard
- Processed Cheese
- Frozen Okra
- Onions
- Peppers (red, green, orange)
- Celery
- Tomatoes
- Parmesan Cheese
- Semi-sweet Chocolate Chips
- Vanilla Extract
- Condensed Milk
- Confectioner's Sugar
- Pork Chops
- Squash
- Spinach
- Cilantro
- Mozzarella Cheese
- Fresh Green Beans

Week 2 Meal Plan

Day One

Total Carb Count: 44g

Breakfast:

Creamy Coconut Porridge (Calories: 322; Fat: 12.4g; Carbohydrates: 5g; Protein: 6g)

Snack

Zoodles Omelet (Calories: 176; Fat: 12.27g; Carbohydrates: 6.2g; Protein: 10.2g)

Lunch

Marinated Shrimp (Calories: 236; Fat: 12g; Carbohydrates: 15g; Protein: 9g)

Snack

Reddy Okra And Tomatoes (Calories: 94; Fat: 4.7g; Carbohydrates: 1.5g; Protein: 3.8g)

Dinner

Portobello Mushroom Burger (Calories: 203 Fat: 14g; Carbohydrates: 9.8g; Protein: 10.3g)

Dessert

Chocolate Truffles (Calories: 53; Fat: 2.5g; Carbohydrates: 7.5g; Protein: 0.9gg)

Day Two

Total Carb Count: 37g

Breakfast:

Creamy Coconut Porridge (Calories: 322; Fat: 12.4g; Carbohydrates: 5g; Protein: 6g)

Snack

Eggplant Tomato (Calories: 55; Fat: 0.38g; Carbohydrates: 9.3g; Protein: 3.3g)

Lunch

Blue Cheese Tenderloin (Calories: 280; Fat; 27g; Carbohydrates: 7g; Protein: 12g)

Snack

Gently Fried Swiss Char (Calories: 56.2; Fat: 3.7g; Carbohydrates: 2.7g; Protein: 39g)

Dinner

Garlic Chicken (Calories: 300 Fat: 16g; Carbohydrates: 5.7g; Protein: 30g)

Dessert

Chocolate Truffles (Calories: 53; Fat: 2.5g; Carbohydrates: 7.5g; Protein: 0.9gg)

Day Three

Total Carb Count: 40.3g

Breakfast:

Coconut Pancakes (Calories: 259; Fat: 15g; Carbohydrates: 6g; Protein: 4g)

Snack

Tender Crisp Broccoli (Calories: 143; Fat: 29.28g; Carbohydrates: 7.6g; Protein: 8.6g)

Lunch

Mushroom Pork Chops (Calories: 210; Fat: 27g; Carbohydrates: 8g; Protein: 23g)

Snack

Reddy Okra And Tomatoes (Calories: 94; Fat: 4.7g; Carbohydrates: 1.5g; Protein: 3.8g)

Dinner

Scrambled Tofu (Calories: 190 Fat: 11.5g; Carbohydrates: 9.7g; Protein: 12g)

Dessert

Chocolate Truffles (Calories: 53; Fat: 2.5g; Carbohydrates: 7.5g; Protein: 0.9gg)

Day Four

Total Carb Count: 33.3g

Breakfast:

Scrambled Eggs (Calories: 317; Fat: 26g; Carbohydrates: 1g; Protein: 19g)

Snack

Tender Crisp Broccoli (Calories: 143; Fat: 29.28g; Carbohydrates: 7.6g; Protein: 8.6g)

Lunch

Blue Cheese Tenderloin (Calories: 280; Fat: 27g; Carbohydrates: 7g; Protein: 12g)

Snack

Roasted Garlic Cauliflower (Calories: 118; Fat: 8.2g; Carbohydrates: 8.6g; Protein: 4.7g)

Dinner

Vegetable Sandwich Spread (Calories: 42 Fat: 3.9g; Carbohydrates: 0.9g; Protein: 1g)

Dessert

Flowerlike Rosettes (Calories: 561; Fat: 59g; Carbohydrates: 8.2g; Protein: 1.1g)

Day Five

Total Carb Count: 32.1

Breakfast:

Creamy Coconut Porridge (Calories: 322; Fat: 12.4g; Carbohydrates: 5g; Protein: 6g)

Snack

Sesame Green Beans (Calories: 333; Fat: 31g; Carbohydrates: 6g; Protein: 7g)

Lunch

Cedar Planked Salmon (Calories: 315; Fat: 15g; Carbohydrates: 10g; Protein: 24g)

Snack

Gently Fried Swiss Chard (Calories: 56.2; Fat: 3.7g; Carbohydrates: 2.7g; Protein: 39g)

Dinner

Vegetable Sandwich Spread (Calories: 42 Fat: 3.9g; Carbohydrates: 0.9g; Protein: 1g)

Dessert

Chocolate Truffles (Calories: 53; Fat: 2.5g; Carbohydrates: 7.5g; Protein: 0.9gg)

Day Six

Total Carb Count: 26g

Breakfast:

Creamy Coconut Porridge (Calories: 322; Fat: 12.4g; Carbohydrates: 5g; Protein: 6g)

Snack

Tender Crisp Broccoli (Calories: 143; Fat: 29.28g; Carbohydrates: 7.6g; Protein: 8.6g)

Lunch

Blue Cheese Tenderloin (Calories: 280; Fat: 27g; Carbohydrates: 7g; Protein: 12g)

Snack

Reddy Okra And Tomatoes (Calories: 94; Fat: 4.7g; Carbohydrates: 1.5g; Protein: 3.8g)

Dinner

Vegetable Sandwich Spread (Calories: 42; Fat: 3.9g; Carbohydrates: 0.9g; Protein: 1g)

Dessert

Creamy Cheese Tart Shells (Calories: 65; Fat: 5g; Carbohydrates: 4g; Protein: 1g)

Day Seven

Total Carb Count: 46.4g

Breakfast:

Creamy Coconut Porridge (Calories: 322; Fat: 12.4g; Carbohydrates: 5g; Protein: 6g)

Snack

Tender Crisp Broccoli (Calories: 143; Fat: 29.28g; Carbohydrates: 7.6g; Protein: 8.6g)

Lunch

Marinated Shrimp (Calories: 236; Fat: 12g; Carbohydrates: 15g; Protein: 9g)

Snack

Reddy Okra And Tomatoes (Calories: 94; Fat: 4.7g: Carbohydrates: 1.5g; Protein: 3.8g)

Dinner

Portobello Mushroom Burger (Calories: 203 Fat: 14g: Carbohydrates: 9.8g; Protein: 10.3g)

Dessert

Chocolate Truffle (Calories: 53; Fat: 2.5g: Carbohydrates: 7.5g; Protein: 0.9gg)

Week 3 Shopping List

- Butter
- Eggs
- Coconut Flour
- Psyllium Husk Powder
- Coconut Cream
- Salt
- Coconut Milk
- Beef Tenderloin
- Teriyaki Sauce
- Red Wine
- Garlic
- Blue Cheese
- Mayonnaise
- Sour Cream
- Worcestershire Sauce
- Oxtail
- Onions
- Seasoning Salt
- Bacon Drippings
- Broth (vegetable, chicken, Beef)
- Garlic Powder
- Salmon
- Black Pepper Corns
- Broccoli Florets

- Dijon Style Mustard
- Processed Cheese
- Frozen Okra
- Peppers (red, green, orange)
- Celery
- Tomatoes
- Parmesan Cheese
- Semi-sweet Chocolate Chips
- Vanilla Extract
- Condensed Milk
- Confectioner's Sugar
- Pork Chops
- Squash
- Spinach
- Cilantro
- Mozzarella Cheese
- Fresh Green Beans
- Tofu
- Shrimp
- Portobello Mushrooms
- Raisins
- Walnuts
- Almonds

Week 3 Meal Plan

Day One

Total Carb Count: 33.3g

Breakfast:

Coconut Pancakes (Calories: 259; Fat: 15g; Carbohydrates: 6g; Protein: 4g)

Snack

Cheesy Tilapia Parmesan (Calories: 224; Fat; 12g; Carbohydrates: 0.8g; Protein: 25.4g)

Lunch

Mushroom Pork Chops (Calories: 210; Fat: 27g; Carbohydrates: 8g; Protein: 23g)

Snack

Reddy Okra And Tomatoes (Calories: 94; Fat: 4.7g; Carbohydrates: 1.5g; Protein: 3.8g)

Dinner

Scrambled Tofu (Calories: 190 Fat: 11.5g; Carbohydrates: 9.7g; Protein: 12g)

Dessert

Chocolate Truffles (Calories: 53; Fat: 2.5g; Carbohydrates: 7.5g; Protein: 0.9gg)

Day Two

Total Carb Count: 35.1g

Breakfast:

Creamy Coconut Porridge (Calories: 322; Fat: 12.4g; Carbohydrates: 5g; Protein: 6g)

Snack

Sesame Green Beans (Calories: 333; Fat: 31g; Carbohydrates: 6g; Protein: 7g)

Lunch

Cedar Planked Salmon (Calories: 315; Fat: 15g; Carbohydrates: 10g; Protein: 24g)

Snack

Gently Fried Swiss Chard (Calories: 56.2; Fat: 3.7g; Carbohydrates: 2.7g; Protein: 39g)

Dinner

Shrimp Etouffé (Calories: 205; Fat: 11g; Carbohydrates: 3.9g; Protein: 22.09g)

Dessert

Chocolate Truffles (Calories: 53; Fat: 2.5g; Carbohydrates: 7.5g; Protein: 0.9gg)

Day Three

Total Carb Count: 60g

Breakfast:

Creamy Coconut Porridge (Calories: 322; Fat: 12.4g; Carbohydrates: 5g; Protein: 6g)

Snack

Tender Crisp Broccoli (Calories: 143; Fat: 29.28g; Carbohydrates: 7.6g; Protein: 8.6g)

Lunch

Marinated Shrimp (Calories: 236; Fat: 12g; Carbohydrates: 15g; Protein: 9g)

Snack

Reddy Okra And Tomatoes (Calories: 94; Fat: 4.7g; Carbohydrates: 1.5g; Protein: 3.8g)

Dinner

Simple BBQ Ribs (Calories: 441; Fat: 22g; Carbohydrates: 24g; Protein: 33g)

Dessert

Chocolate Truffles (Calories: 53; Fat: 2.5g; Carbohydrates: 7.5g; Protein: 0.9gg)

Day Four

Total Carb Count: 16.1g

Breakfast:

Creamy Coconut Porridge (Calories: 322; Fat: 12.4g: Carbohydrates: 5g; Protein: 6g)

Snack

Prosciutto Wrapped Asparagus (Calories: 56; Fat: 3.6g: Carbohydrates: 2.7g; Protein: 39g)

Lunch

Blue Cheese Tenderloin (Calories: 280; Fat: 27g: Carbohydrates: 7g; Protein: 12g)

Snack

Reddy Okra And Tomatoes (Calories: 94; Fat: 4.7g: Carbohydrates: 1.5g; Protein: 3.8g)

Dinner

Vegetable Sandwich Spread (Calories: 42 Fat: 3.9g: Carbohydrates: 0.9g; Protein: 1g)

Dessert

Creamy Cheese Tart Shells (Calories: 65; Fat: 5g: Carbohydrates: 4g; Protein: 1g)

Day Five

Total Carb Count: 35.1g

Breakfast:

Scrambled Eggs (Calories: 317; Fat: 26g: Carbohydrates: 1g; Protein: 19g)

Snack

Tender Crisp Broccoli (Calories: 143; Fat: 29.28g: Carbohydrates: 7.6g; Protein: 8.6g)

Lunch

Blue Cheese Tenderloin (Calories: 280; Fat: 27g: Carbohydrates: 7g; Protein: 12g)

Snack

Roasted Garlic Cauliflower (Calories: 118; Fat: 8.2g: Carbohydrates: 8.6g; Protein: 4.7g)

Dinner

Vegetable Sandwich Spread (Calories: 42 Fat: 3.9g: Carbohydrates: 0.9g; Protein: 1g)

Dessert

Sticky Ganache (Calories: 172; Fat: 13g: Carbohydrates: 10g; Protein: 1.5g)

Day Six

Total Carb Count: 40g

Breakfast:

Creamy Coconut Porridge (Calories: 322; Fat: 12.4g: Carbohydrates: 5g; Protein: 6g)

Snack

Zoodles Omelet (Calories: 176; Fat: 12.27g: Carbohydrates: 6.2g; Protein: 10.2g)

Lunch

Marinated Shrimp (Calories: 236; Fat: 12g: Carbohydrates: 15g; Protein: 9g)

Snack

Reddy Okra And Tomatoes (Calories: 94; Fat: 4.7g: Carbohydrates: 1.5g; Protein: 3.8g)

Dinner

Portobello Mushroom Burger (Calories: 203 Fat: 14g: Carbohydrates: 9.8g; Protein: 10.3g)

Dessert

Raw Candy (Calories: 45; Fat: 3.5g: Carbohydrates: 3.2g; Protein: 1g)

Day Seven

Total Carb Count: 46.8g

Breakfast:

Coconut Pancakes (Calories: 259; Fat: 15g: Carbohydrates: 6g; Protein: 4g)

Snack

Tender Crisp Broccoli (Calories: 143; Fat: 29.28g: Carbohydrates: 7.6g; Protein: 8.6g)

Lunch

Marinated Shrimp (Calories: 236; Fat: 12g: Carbohydrates: 15g; Protein: 9g)

Snack

Reddy Okra And Tomatoes (Calories: 94; Fat: 4.7g: Carbohydrates: 1.5g; Protein: 3.8g)

Dinner

Portobello Mushroom Burger (Calories: 203 Fat: 14g: Carbohydrates: 9.8g; Protein: 10.3g)

Dessert

Chocolate Truffles (Calories: 53; Fat: 2.5g: Carbohydrates: 7.5g; Protein: 0.9gg)

Week 4 Shopping List

- Butter
- Eggs
- Coconut Flour
- Psyllium Husk Powder
- Coconut Cream
- Salt
- Coconut Milk
- Beef Tenderloin
- Teriyaki Sauce
- Red Wine
- Garlic
- Blue Cheese
- Mayonnaise
- Sour Cream
- Worcestershire Sauce
- Oxtail
- Onions
- Seasoning Salt
- Bacon Drippings
- Broth (vegetable, chicken, beef)
- Garlic Powder
- Salmon
- Black Pepper Corns
- Broccoli Florets

- Dijon Style Mustard
- Processed Cheese
- Frozen Okra
- Peppers (red, green, orange)
- Celery
- Tomatoes
- Parmesan Cheese
- Semi-sweet Chocolate Chips
- Vanilla Extract
- Condensed Milk
- Confectioner's Sugar
- Pork Chops
- Squash
- Spinach
- Cilantro
- Mozzarella Cheese
- Fresh Green Beans
- Tofu
- Shrimp
- Portobello Mushrooms
- Raisins
- Walnuts
- Almonds

Week 4 Meal Plan

Day One

Total Carb Count: 40g

Breakfast:

Creamy Coconut Porridge (Calories: 322; Fat: 12.4g: Carbohydrates: 5g; Protein: 6g)

Snack

Zoodles Omelet (Calories: 176; Fat: 12.27g: Carbohydrates: 6.2g; Protein: 10.2g)

Lunch

Marinated Shrimp (Calories: 236; Fat: 12g: Carbohydrates: 15g; Protein: 9g)

Snack

Reddy Okra And Tomatoes (Calories: 94; Fat: 4.7g: Carbohydrates: 1.5g; Protein: 3.8g)

Dinner

Portobello Mushroom Burger (Calories: 203 Fat: 14g: Carbohydrates: 9.8g; Protein: 10.3g)

Dessert

Raw Candy (Calories: 45; Fat: 3.5g: Carbohydrates: 3.2g; Protein: 1g)

Day Two

Total Carb Count: 26g

Breakfast:

Creamy Coconut Porridge (Calories: 322; Fat: 12.4g: Carbohydrates: 5g; Protein: 6g)

Snack

Tender Crisp Broccoli (Calories: 143; Fat: 29.28g: Carbohydrates: 7.6g; Protein: 8.6g)

Lunch

Blue Cheese Tenderloin (Calories: 280; Fat: 27g: Carbohydrates: 7g; Protein: 12g)

Snack

Reddy Okra And Tomatoes (Calories: 94; Fat: 4.7g: Carbohydrates: 1.5g; Protein: 3.8g)

Dinner

Vegetable Sandwich Spread (Calories: 42 Fat: 3.9g: Carbohydrates: 0.9g; Protein: 1g)

Dessert

Creamy Cheese Tart Shells (Calories: 65; Fat: 5g: Carbohydrates: 4g; Protein: 1g)

Day Three

Total Carb Count: 33.3g

Breakfast:

Scrambled Eggs (Calories: 317; Fat: 26g: Carbohydrates: 1g; Protein: 19g)

Snack

Tender Crisp Broccoli (Calories: 143; Fat: 29.28g: Carbohydrates: 7.6g; Protein: 8.6g)

Lunch

Blue Cheese Tenderloin (Calories: 280; Fat: 27g: Carbohydrates: 7g; Protein: 12g)

Snack

Roasted Garlic Cauliflower (Calories: 118; Fat: 8.2g: Carbohydrates: 8.6g; Protein: 4.7g)

Dinner

Vegetable Sandwich Spread (Calories: 42 Fat: 3.9g: Carbohydrates: 0.9g; Protein: 1g)

Dessert

Flowerlike Rosettes (Calories: 561; Fat: 59g: Carbohydrates: 8.2g; Protein: 1.1g)

Day Four

Total Carb Count: 37g

Breakfast:

Creamy Coconut Porridge (Calories: 322; Fat: 12.4g: Carbohydrates: 5g; Protein: 6g)

Snack

Baked Eggplant Tomato (Calories: 55; Fat: 0.38g: Carbohydrates: 9.3g; Protein: 3.3g)

Lunch

Blue Cheese Tenderloin (Calories: 280; Fat: 27g: Carbohydrates: 7g; Protein: 12g)

Snack

Gently Fried Swiss Char (Calories: 56.2; Fat: 3.7g: Carbohydrates: 2.7g; Protein: 39g)

Dinner

Garlic Chicken (Calories: 300 Fat: 16g: Carbohydrates: 5.7g; Protein: 30g)

Dessert

Chocolate Truffles (Calories: 53; Fat: 2.5g: Carbohydrates: 7.5g; Protein: 0.9gg)

Day Five

Total Carb Count: 39.3g

Breakfast:

Coconut Pancakes (Calories: 259; Fat: 15g: Carbohydrates: 6g; Protein: 4g)

Snack

Tender Crisp Broccoli (Calories: 143; Fat: 29.28g: Carbohydrates: 7.6g; Protein: 8.6g)

Lunch

Blue Cheese Tenderloin (Calories: 280; Fat: 27g: Carbohydrates: 7g; Protein: 12g)

Snack

Reddy Okra And Tomatoes (Calories: 94; Fat: 4.7g: Carbohydrates: 1.5g; Protein: 3.8g)

Dinner

Scrambled Tofu (Calories: 190 Fat: 11.5g: Carbohydrates: 9.7g; Protein: 12g)

Dessert

Chocolate Truffles (Calories: 53; Fat: 2.5g: Carbohydrates: 7.5g; Protein: 0.9gg)

Day Six

Total Carb Count: 32g

Breakfast:

Creamy Coconut Porridge (Calories: 322; Fat: 12.4g: Carbohydrates: 5g; Protein: 6g)

Snack

Baked Eggplant Tomato (Calories: 55; Fat: 0.38g: Carbohydrates: 9.3g; Protein: 3.3g)

Lunch

Blue Cheese Tenderloin (Calories: 280; Fat: 27g: Carbohydrates: 7g; Protein: 12g)

Snack

Gently Fried Swiss Char (Calories: 56.2; Fat: 3.7g: Carbohydrates: 2.7g; Protein: 39g)

Dinner

Vegetable Sandwich Spread (Calories: 42 Fat: 3.9g: Carbohydrates: 0.9g; Protein: 1g)

Dessert

Chocolate Truffles (Calories: 53; Fat: 2.5g: Carbohydrates: 7.5g; Protein: 0.9gg)

Day Seven

Total Carb Count: 46.4g

Breakfast:

Creamy Coconut Porridge (Calories: 322; Fat: 12.4g: Carbohydrates: 5g; Protein: 6g)

Snack

Tender Crisp Broccoli (Calories: 143; Fat: 29.28g: Carbohydrates: 7.6g; Protein: 8.6g)

Lunch

Marinated Shrimp (Calories: 236; Fat: 12g: Carbohydrates: 15g; Protein: 9g)

Snack

Reddy Okra And Tomatoes (Calories: 94; Fat: 4.7g: Carbohydrates: 1.5g; Protein: 3.8g)

Dinner

Portobello Mushroom Burger (Calories: 203 Fat: 14g: Carbohydrates: 9.8g; Protein: 10.3g)

Dessert

Chocolate Truffles (Calories: 53; Fat: 2.5g: Carbohydrates: 7.5g; Protein: 0.9gg)

Chapter 5: Delicious Breakfasts

1. Creamy Coconut Porridge

(Prep time: 5 minutes\ Cook time: 10 minutes\ Serving: 1)

Ingredients:

- 1 teaspoon of butter
- 1 egg
- 1 Tablespoon coconut flour
- Pinch of ground psyllium husk powder
- 4 Tablespoons coconut cream
- Pinch of salt

Directions:

1) In a small saucepan, melt the butter.
2) Add the coconut flour, husk powder, pinch of salt. Whisk together.
3) Cook for 2-4 minutes until desired consistency is reached.
4) Pour in a bowl. Top with coconut cream, and fresh berries.

Nutrition Value:

- Calories: 322
- Fat: 124g
- Carbohydrates: 5g
- Protein: 6g
- Dietary Fiber: 4.2g

2. Scrambled Egg

(Prep time: 5 minutes\ Cook time: 5 minutes\ Serving: 1)

Ingredients:

- 3 large eggs
- 2 teaspoons butter
- Salt and fresh ground pepper to taste
- Garnish: chives

Directions:

1) In a small bowl, crack all the eggs.
2) Whisk the eggs until they turn a pale yellow. Sprinkle in salt and pepper.
3) In a medium frying pan, over medium heat, melt the butter.
4) Pour in the egg mixture.
5) Using a spatula, stir the eggs constantly, until they form a creamy texture.
6) Plate and serve immediately. Optional: garnish with chives.

Nutrition Value

- Calories: 317
- Fat: 26g
- Carbohydrates: 1g
- Protein: 19g

3. Coconut Pancakes

(Prep time: 5 minutes\ Cook time: 30 minutes\ Servings: 4)

Ingredients:

- 6 eggs
- ½ cup coconut flour
- ¾ cup coconut milk
- 2 Tablespoons coconut oil, melted
- 1 teaspoon baking powder
- Pinch of salt
- 1–2 teaspoons butter
- Fresh berries

Directions:

1) You will need two bowls. Separate the egg whites and yolks.
2) Using a whisk or hand blender, blend the egg whites until soft peaks form.
3) In the other bowl, add the oil and coconut milk to the egg yolks. Mix well.
4) In the same bowl, add the flour, baking powder and salt. Mix until combined.

5) Fold the egg whites into your batter. Let it stand for 5 minutes.
6) In a large frying pan, melt the butter. Using an ice cream scoop, ladle pancake mix in the frying pan.
7) Cook for 1-2 minutes until bubbles form on the top. Flip, cook the other side.
8) Serve immediately. Side with fresh berries.

Nutrition Value

- Calories: 259
- Fat: 15g
- Carbohydrates: 6g
- Protein: 4g

4. Devilled Eggs

(Prep time: 5 minutes\ Cook time: 10 minutes\ Servings: 4)

Ingredients:

- 8 eggs
- ¼ cup mayonnaise
- Garnish: chives

Directions:

1) In a large pot, place all the eggs.
2) Fill the pot with cold water until the eggs are covered.
3) Bring the water to a boil.
4) Boil for 10 minutes. Turn heat off. Leave the pot on element for 10 minutes.
5) Dump the water. Run cold water over the eggs. Peel the shells, rinse in clean, cold water.
6) Slice the eggs in half. Pop the yellows into a bowl. Break them up. Cool for 10 minutes.
7) Mash up the yolk. Add mayonnaise. Mix well.

8) Using a spoon, fill the halves with the egg mixture.
9) Garnish with chives.
10)　　Serve immediately or chill until ready to eat.

Nutrition Value

- Calories: 109
- Fat: 7g
- Carbohydrates: 4g
- Protein: 9g

5. Healthy Salad Sandwich

(Prep time: 2 minutes\ Cook time: 2 minutes\ Servings: 4)

Ingredients:

- 3 large pieces of lettuce, your choice
- 2 pieces cooked lean meat, your choice, diced
- ¼ cup cheese, medium or sharp cheddar, grated
- ½ an avocado, diced
- Dressing, a light vinaigrette
- 1 tomato, diced

Directions:

1) Rinse your letter and pat dry.
2) In a medium bowl, combine the meat, avocado, cheese, and tomato.
3) Pour in the dressing. Toss until all ingredients coated.
4) Plate the lettuce.
5) Scoop the ingredients over the lettuce leafs.

- Serve immediately.

Nutrition Value:

- Calories: 262
- Fat: 12g
- Carbohydrates: 10g
- Protein: 14g

6. Warm Egg Muffins

(Prep time: 5 minutes\ Cook time: 20 minutes\ Servings: 4)

Ingredients:

- 6 egg
- 1-2 shallots, finely chopped
- 4-8 slices bacon, cooked
- ½ cup shredded cheese
- 1 Tablespoon salsa
- Pinch of salt and fresh ground pepper, each
- Muffin tin
- Oil to coat muffin tins

Directions:

1) Preheat oven to 375°F.
2) Chop up the cooked bacon and shallots.
3) In a large bowl, crack the eggs. Add the salt and pepper, salsa, crumbled bacon and cheese. Mix until combined.
4) Pour the batter in the muffin tins, ¾ full.

5) Bake for 15-20 minutes, or until golden brown.
6) Serve immediately.

Nutrition Value:

- Calories: 92
- Fat: 5g
- Carbohydrates: 7g
- Protein: 4g

7. Banana Waffles

(Prep time: 10 minutes\ Cook time: 20 minutes\ Servings: 8)

Ingredients:

- 2 ripe bananas, mashed
- 4 eggs
- ¼ cup almond milk
- ½ teaspoon vanilla extract
- 1 Tablespoon ground psyllium husk powder or 1 Tablespoon almond flour
- 1 teaspoon baking powder
- 1 teaspoon ground cinnamon
- Coconut oil or butter to coat waffle maker

Directions:

1) In a medium bowl, combine the dry ingredients.
2) Add the mashed bananas, eggs, almond milk, and vanilla extract. Mix well.
3) Preheat your waffle maker. Coat with oil or butter. Spoon the batter to just before

the edge of the grill. Close and cook 3 – 5 minutes, or until golden brown.

4) Serve immediately. Side with fresh berries.

Nutrition Value:

- Calories: 120
- Fat: 7g
- Carbohydrates: 15g
- Protein: 2g

8. Eggplant Hash With Eggs

(Prep time: 10 minutes\ Cook time: 10 minutes\ Servings: 4)

Ingredients:

- 4-8 eggs
- 1 small eggplant
- 2 Tablespoons flavorless oil, your choice
- ¼ cup mozzarella cheese, cubed
- ½ onion, diced
- 2 Tablespoons butter
- 8-10 cherry tomatoes, halved
- 1 Tablespoon vinegar
- Garnish: Worcestershire sauce

Directions:

1) Dice the eggplant. Dice the onion. Cube the cheese.
2) In a large frying pan, heat the oil. Add the onions. Sweat them for 2 minutes.
3) Add the egg plant. Cook for 5 minutes, until it becomes fork tender.

4) Season with salt and pepper. Add the cherry tomatoes.
5) Bring a medium pot with 6 cups of water to boil. Add 1 tablespoon of vinegar. Crack 1 egg at a time. Cook to desired consistency.
6) Add the cubed cheese to the eggplant as the eggs cook.
7) Plate the eggplant. Top with eggs. Garnish with Worcestershire sauce.

Nutrition Value:

- Calories: 280
- Fat: 27g
- Carbohydrates: 7g
- Protein: 12g

Chapter 6: Appetizing Lunches

9. Blue Cheese Beef Tenderloin

(Prep time: 30 minutes\ Cook time: 60 minutes\ Servings: 8)

Ingredients:

- 3 pound (whole piece) beef tenderloin
- ½ cup red wine
- ½ cup teriyaki sauce
- 2 garlic cloves, chopped
- ½ cup blue cheese, crumbled
- ⅓ cup mayonnaise
- ⅔ cup of sour cream
- 1 ½ cups Worcestershire sauce

Directions:

1) In a bowl, combine the red wine, teriyaki sauce, and garlic.
2) Place the tenderloin in a baking dish. Pour the marinade over the beef. Turn the tenderloin around in the dish, coating all sides.
3) Cover the baking dish. Refrigerate 30 minutes.

4) Preheat oven to 450°F.
5) Remove plastic from baking dish. Place in the oven. Cook at 450°F for 15 minutes.
6) Turn down the oven temperature to 375°degrees. Cook for 30-40 minutes.
7) Take the tenderloin out of the oven. Place it on a platter. Let it rest for 10 minutes.
8) Place the baking dish on an element, low heat. Add the blue cheese, mayonnaise, sour cream, and Worcestershire sauce. Mix until combined and smooth.
9) Slice the tenderloin. Place on a platter. Drizzle cheese sauce over tenderloin.
10)   Serve with a side of white or brown rice, salad.

Nutrition Value:

- Calories: 219
- Fat: 8.3g
- Carbohydrates: 1g
- Protein: 32g

10. Juicy Oxtail with Gravy

(Prep time: 10 minutes\ Cook time: 3 hours 20 minutes\ Servings: 6)

Ingredients:

- 2 pounds of oxtail, cubed
- 1 garlic clove, minced
- 1 onion, diced
- 1 Tablespoon Greek seasoning
- 1 teaspoon seasoning salt
- 2 Tablespoon bacon drippings
- 2 Tablespoons all-purpose flour
- Worcestershire sauce
- Pinch of salt and fresh ground pepper, each
- Pinch of garlic powder

Directions:

1) In a large stock pot, heat up the oil. Add the diced onion. Sweat them for 2 minutes. Add the minced garlic. Cook for 1 minute.

2) Place the pieces of oxtail in the pot. Sear on all sides.
3) Add salt, pepper, and Greek seasoning.
4) Fill the pot with water to cover the pieces of oxtail.
5) Bring the mixture to a boil. Reduce the temperature. Cover and simmer for 3 hours.
6) Remove from the heat. Reserve 2 cups of the broth.
7) Using the same pot, on high heat, add the flour and cook for 1-2 minutes, stirring constantly, add a bit of the warm oxtail broth, keep stirring until combined. Pour in the rest or the broth.
8) Place the cooked oxtail in the gravy. Simmer for 5 minutes over low heat.
9) Serve immediately. Side with salad or potatoes.

Nutrition Value:

- Calories: 234
- Fat: 35g
- Carbohydrates: 15g
- Protein: 24g

11. Cedar Planked Salmon

(Prep time: 25 minutes\ Cook time: 15 minutes\ Servings: 6)

Ingredients:

- 24x8x1 inch of untreated cider plank
- 6 ounce piece of salmon, skin on
- ½ cup flavorless oil, your choice
- 1 large red onion, sliced
- 1 lemon, sliced
- ½ Tablespoon fresh ground pepper

Directions:

1) Submerge your untreated cedar plank in water. Soak overnight.
2) Preheat your outdoor grill at high heat.
3) Place your prepared plank on your grill. Sprinkle it with salt.
4) Close the grill and heat up the plank for 2-3 minutes.
5) Reduce the temperature to medium heat.
6) Rub the salmon fillet with your choice of oil. Place it on the plank.

7) Grind pepper over the salmon. Cover the salmon with sliced onion, lemon slices.
8) Close the lid of the grill. Cook the salmon for 10-12 minutes, until salmon is flaky.
9) Serve immediately. Side with white or brown rice, salad.

Nutrition Value:

- Calories: 241
- Fat: 11g
- Carbohydrates: 0g
- Protein: 34g

12. Marinated Shrimp

(Prep time: 30 minutes\ Cook time: 10 minutes\ Servings: 6)

Ingredients:

- 2 pounds fresh shrimp, deveined
- ¼ cup fresh parsley, chopped
- Juice squeezed from 1 lemon
- 2 Tablespoons hot sauce
- 3 garlic cloves, minced
- 1 Tablespoon tomato paste
- 2 teaspoons dried oregano
- 1 teaspoon salt
- 1 teaspoon fresh ground pepper
- Oil for basting the grill

Directions:

1) Rinse the shrimp and pat dry.
2) Combine all the ingredients in a large baggie, and 1 tablespoon of the oil. Don't add the shrimp yet. Massage the bag until the ingredients are combined.

3) Add the shrimp. Squeeze the bag until all the shrimp are coated.
4) Place in refrigerator. Marinate for 2 hours.
5) After 2 hours, thread the shrimp on skewers. Discard the remaining marinade.
6) Preheat your grill to medium-low heat.
7) Lightly oil the grill. Place skewers on the grill. Cook the shrimp 5 minutes per side.
8) Serve immediately. Side with salad.

Nutrition Value:

- Calories: 236
- Fat: 12g
- Carbohydrates: 15g
- Protein: 9g

13. Portobello Mushroom Burger

(Prep time 15 minutes\ Cook time: 20 minutes\ Servings: 4)

Ingredients:

- 4 Portobello mushroom caps
- ¼ cup balsamic vinegar
- 2 Tablespoons flavorless oil, your choice
- 1 teaspoon dried basil
- 1 teaspoon dried oregano
- 1 garlic clove, minced
- Pinch of salt and fresh ground pepper, each
- 4 slices provolone cheese
- 4 whole wheat buns

Directions:

1) Rinse the mushroom caps, pat dry.
2) In a small bowl, combine the vinegar, oil, basil, oregano, garlic, salt and pepper.
3) Pour the mix over your mushrooms.
4) Marinate in the sauce for 15 minutes. Turn every 5 minutes.

5) Preheat your grill to medium-high heat.
6) Brush grill with oil.
7) Place your mushrooms on the grill. Reserve the marinade for basting.
8) Cook for 5-8 minutes per side. Brush with the marinade.
9) Place the buns on the grill, low heat.
10) Top the mushrooms with cheese during final minute on the grill.
11) Serve hot. Side with salad.

Nutrition Value:

- Calories: 203
- Fat: 14g
- Carbohydrates: 9.8g
- Protein: 10.3g

14. Scrambled Tofu

(Prep time: 10 minutes\ Cook time: 15 minutes\ Servings: 4)

Ingredients:

- 12 ounce package Tofu, drained and diced
- 1 Tablespoon flavorless oil
- 2 stocks green onion, diced
- 1 large can tomatoes, peeled and diced with juice
- Pinch of ground turmeric
- Pinch of salt and fresh ground pepper, each
- Garnish: cheddar cheese, grated

Directions:

1) In a medium skillet, heat the oil over medium heat.
2) Add the green onions, sweat for 1 minute.
3) Stir in the tomatoes, and diced tofu.
4) Season with turmeric, salt and pepper.

5) Cover, reduce the heat. Simmer until the tofu is tender.
6) Serve immediately. Garnish with grated cheese.

Nutrition Value:

- Calories: 190
- Fat: 11.5g
- Carbohydrates: 9.7g
- Protein: 12g

15. Broiled Cheesy Tilapia Parmesan

(Prep time: 15 minutes\ Cook time: 10 minutes\ Servings: 8)

Ingredients:

- 2 pounds tilapia fillets
- ½ cup parmesan cheese
- ¼ cup butter
- 1 Tablespoon fresh squeezed lemon juice
- 3 Tablespoons mayonnaise
- 2 Tablespoons fresh ground pepper
- ⅛ teaspoon onion powder
- ⅛ teaspoon celery salt

Directions:

1) Rinse the tilapia, pat dry. Season with salt, pepper, onion powder, celery salt.
2) In a small bowl, combine the parmesan cheese, butter, mayonnaise, lemon juice.
3) Preheat broiler in your oven.
4) Arrange the fillets in a single layer on baking pan.

5) Broil a few inches from heat source for 3 minutes, flip and broil for 2 minutes.
6) Remove the fillets, pour the parmesan cheese mix over the fillets.
7) Return to broiler for 2 minutes, until topping is golden browned.
8) Serve immediately. Side with white or brown rice, salad.

Nutrition Value:

- Calories: 224
- Fat: 12g
- Carbohydrates: 0.8g
- Protein: 25.4g

16. Shrimp Etouffé

(Prep time: 30 minutes\ Cook time: 1 hour 45 minutes\ Servings: 10)

Ingredients:

- 5 pounds fresh shrimp, deveined, tails removed
- 1 cup of butter
- 2 large white onions, diced
- 6 stalks of celery, diced
- 3 garlic cloves, minced
- 4 Tablespoons all-purpose flour
- 2 cups + ¼ cup water
- 3 Tablespoons paprika
- Pinch of salt and fresh ground pepper, each
- Pinch crushed chili flakes

Directions:

1) Rinse the shrimp, pat dry.
2) In a large skillet, melt the butter.
3) Add the onions, garlic, and celery. Sauté for 5 minutes.

4) Add the shrimp. Cook for 5 minutes, or until the shrimp turn pink.
5) In a small cup, combine the flour and ¼ cup water. Mix until it forms a slurry (thickening agent for the dish). Set aside.
6) Add 2 cups water to skillet. Stir in paprika, salt, pepper, crushed chili. Mix well.
7) Stir in slurry mixture. Cook for 5 minutes, until it thickens.
8) Serve immediately. Side with white or brown rice, salad.

Nutrition Value:

- Calories: 205
- Fat: 11g
- Carbohydrates: 3.9g
- Protein: 22.9g

Chapter 7: Mouth-Watering Dinners

17. Vegetable Sandwich Spread

(Prep time: 30 minutes\ Cook time: 1 hour 49 minutes\ Servings: 10)

Ingredients:

- 8 ounce cream cheese, room temperature
- 1 ½ cup shredded carrots
- 1 ½ cup shredded zucchini
- 1 ½ Tablespoon fresh parsley, chopped
- ½ teaspoon garlic powder
- Pinch of salt and fresh ground pepper, each
- Pinch of paprika
- Pinch of garlic salt

Directions:

1) In a medium-sized bowl, blend the cream cheese until smooth.
2) Add the zucchini, carrot, garlic powder, parsley, onion powder, paprika, pepper, and garlic salt. Stir until combined.
3) Cover. Place in refrigerator. Chill for 30 minutes.

4) Serve as a dinner side or spread on your favorite sandwich.

Nutrition Value:

- Calories: 42
- Fat: 3.9g
- Carbohydrates: 0.9g
- Protein: 1g

18. Zoodles Omelet

(Prep time: 10 minutes\ Cook time: 15 minutes\ Servings: 2)

Ingredients:

- 1 yellow squash
- 1 Tablespoon of butter
- ¼ cup fresh spinach
- 2 Tablespoons fresh cilantro, chopped
- 2 eggs
- ¼ cup milk
- ¼ cup mozzarella cheese, grated
- Pinch of salt and fresh ground pepper, each

Directions:

1) Slice off the bulbous, seeded end of the squash. Slice off shorter end.
2) Peel the squash completely. Cut the squash in half.
3) Align the first piece of squash on spiralizer. Turn the handle, spiralize the squash.

4) Heat up a large skillet over medium heat. Melt the butter.
5) Toss in squash zoodles, cilantro, and spinach.
6) Cook 5-7 minutes, until tender.
7) In a small bowl, combine the eggs and milk.
8) Pour over the squash mixture. Stir until noodles are coated.
9) Cook until the egg is gently firm, approximately 5 minutes.
10)   Sprinkle the mozzarella cheese over the mixture. Heat until the cheese is melted.
11) Serve immediately.

Nutrition Value:

- Calories: 176
- Fat: 12.7g
- Carbohydrates: 6.2g
- Protein: 10.2g

19. Chicken Curry Salad

(Prep time: 5 minutes\ Cook time: 20 minutes\ Servings: 8)

Ingredients:

- 4 chicken breasts, skinless, boneless
- 1 teaspoon flavorless oil, your choice
- ¼ cup golden raisins
- ⅓ cup seedless green grapes
- ½ cup toasted pecans, chopped
- ⅛ teaspoon fresh ground pepper
- ½ teaspoon curry powder
- 1 stalk of celery, chopped
- ½ white onion, diced
- 1 small green apple, peeled, cubed
- ¾ cup mayonnaise, hellman's
- ¼ cup white wine

Directions:

1) Rinse the chicken, pat dry.
2) In a large frying pan, heat up the oil. Cook the chicken, season with salt and

pepper. Once cooked, cut into cubes. Cool in refrigerator as you prepare the rest.

3) In a large bowl, combine the onion, celery, apple, raisins, pepper, pecans, curry powder, white wine, and mayonnaise. Stir until combined.

4) Add the chicken. Stir until chicken is coated.

5) Serve immediately.

Nutrition Value:

- Calories: 306
- Fat: 23g
- Carbohydrates: 11.5g
- Protein: 15g

20. Garlic Chicken

(Prep time: 20 minutes\ Cook time: 35 minutes\ Servings: 2)

Ingredients:

- 2 chicken legs, 2 chicken thighs
- 1 egg
- ¼ cup flavorless oil, your choice
- 2 garlic cloves, crushed
- ¼ cup Italian bread crumbs
- ¼ cup parmesan cheese, grated
- 6-8 cherry tomatoes, halved

Directions:

1) Rinse the chicken, pat dry.
2) Preheat oven to 425°F.
3) In a large skillet, heat the oil.
4) You will need 2 bowls. One for the egg. One for the bread crumbs.
5) Dip the chicken in the egg first. Then the bread crumbs.
6) Fry the chicken in the oil, 4-6 minutes on each side.

7) Transfer the chicken to a shallow baking dish. Sprinkle the parmesan cheese over the chicken. Place the tomatoes in the dish. Drizzle a bit more oil over the tomatoes.
8) Bake for 30-35 minutes.
9) Serve immediately. Side with whole wheat pasta, salad.

Nutrition Value:

- Calories: 300
- Fat: 16g
- Carbohydrates: 5.7g
- Protein: 30g

21. Simple BBQ Ribs

(Prep time: 30 minutes\ Cook time: 90 minutes\ Servings: 4)

Ingredients:

- 2 ½ pounds country-style pork ribs
- 1 Tablespoon garlic powder
- 1 teaspoon fresh ground pepper
- 2 Tablespoons salt
- 1 cup barbeque sauce

Directions:

1) It might be easier to chop the ribs into sections. Rinse them and pat dry.
2) In a large stock pot, place the ribs. Fill with water until the meat is covered.
3) Season the water and ribs with the salt, pepper, and garlic powder.
4) Bring the water to a low boil. Cover and cook the ribs until they are just tender, approximately 45 minutes.
5) Preheat oven to 325°F.
6) Remove the ribs from the pot, place them in a shallow baking dish.

7) Pour barbecue sauce over the ribs, turn them over, and coat other side.
8) Cover with aluminum foil. Bake for 1 ½ hours, turn ribs halfway through cooking.
9) Take the foil off last 5 minutes, pour more barbecue sauce on the ribs. Broil 2 minutes per side to create a crust.
10)   Serve immediately. Side with salad.

Nutrition Value:

- Calories: 441
- Fat: 22g
- Carbohydrates: 24g
- Protein: 33g

22. Mushroom Pork Chops

(Prep time: 10 minutes\ Cook time: 30 minutes\ Servings: 4)

Ingredients:

- 4 butterfly pork chops
- 1 teaspoon flavorless oil, your choice
- Pinch of salt and fresh ground pepper, each
- Pinch of garlic salt
- 1 onion, chopped
- ½ pound fresh mushrooms, diced
- 1 can condensed cream of mushroom soup
- 2 Tablespoons low-sodium beef broth

Directions:

1) Rinse your pork chops, pat dry.
2) Season both sides with salt, pepper and garlic salt.
3) In a large frying pan, heat the oil and add the onions. Let them sweat for 2 minutes (they will turn translucent).

4) Place the pork chops in the frying pan. Cook on each side for 8-10 minutes.
5) Add the mushrooms to the pan. Sauté them for 1 minute.
6) Pull the pork chops out of the pan, place on a plate. Pour the condensed soup into frying pan over the mushrooms. Add the beef broth. Turn the heat to medium-high. Stir the mixture until it becomes smooth.
7) Return pork chops to pan. Coat with the soup. Simmer on low for 10 minutes.
8) Serve immediately. Side with a salad.

Nutrition Value:
- Calories: 210
- Fat: 8g
- Carbohydrates: 9.6g
- Protein: 23g

23. Cheesy Pork Chops

(Prep time: 10 minutes\ Cook time: 20 minutes\ Servings: 4)

Ingredients:

- 4 butterfly pork chops
- 1 Tablespoon flavorless oil, your choice
- Juice squeezed from 1-2 lemons (enough to dip each pork chop)
- ½ white onion, diced
- 1 garlic clove, minced
- 1 teaspoon dry rosemary
- 1 teaspoon dried basil
- Pinch of fresh ground pepper
- ½-1 cup Monterey jack cheese, grated

Directions:

1) Rinse your pork chops, pat dry.
2) In a large skillet, heat the oil. Add the diced onion. Sweat for 2 minutes. Add the garlic. Cook for 1 minute.

3) Dip the pork chops in the lemon juice. Season both sides of the pork chops with rosemary, basil, and pepper.
4) Place them in the frying pan, sear each side to create a crust.
5) Cover the pan, reduce to medium heat. Cook for another 8-10 minutes, until middle is cooked.
6) Sprinkle with the grated cheese. Cover the pan to let the cheese melt.
7) Serve immediately. Side with green beans.

Nutrition Value:

- Calories: 316
- Fat: 21g
- Carbohydrates: 6g
- Protein: 25g

24. Slightly Tangy Baked Soy Lemon Chops

(Prep time: 15 minutes\ Cook time: 40 minutes\ Servings: 4)

Ingredients:

- 4 butterfly pork chops
- ½ cup soy sauce
- 1 Tablespoon Worcestershire sauce
- 4 garlic cloves, minced
- 2 Tablespoons lemon juice
- ½ teaspoon flavorless oil, your choice

Directions:

1) Rinse the pork chops, pat dry.
2) In a shallow glass dish, combine the soy sauce, Worcestershire sauce, lemon juice, garlic, pepper and oil. Stir gently to combine.
3) Dip the pork chops in the marinade, turning a few times to coat completely. Cover with plastic wrap, refrigerate for 1 hour.

4) When ready to cook them, preheat oven to 375°F.
5) Place your marinated chops in a shallow baking dish. Bake for 35-40 minutes, until middle is cooked (internal temperature 145°F).
6) Serve immediately. Side with a salad or a cooked, green vegetable.

Nutrition Value:

- Calories: 193
- Fat: 6g
- Carbohydrates: 5g
- Protein: 27g

Chapter 8:
Fulfilling
Snacks

25. Tender Crisp Broccoli

(Prep time: 10 minutes\ Cook time: 10 minutes\ Servings: 4)

Ingredients:

- 1 large broccoli, cut into florets
- 2 Tablespoons kosher salt (for cooking florets)
- 1 Tablespoon flavorless oil
- 1/2-1 teaspoon lemon juice
- 1 garlic clove, minced
- Pinch of salt and fresh ground pepper, each

Directions:

1) Place the florets in a large stock pot. Cover the florets with water.
2) Pour in the salt.
3) Bring the broccoli to a boil. Cook for 1 minute.
4) Dump the florets in a colander (strainer) and place the colander into an ice bath. (This stops the cooking process.)

5) Place the florets back in the pot. Toss the florets with oil, lemon juice, salt, pepper, and garlic.
6) Serve immediately.

Nutrition Value:

- Calories. 150
- Fat: 11g
- Carbohydrates: 12g
- Protein: 5g

26. Reddy Okra And Tomatoes

(Prep time: 10 minutes\ Cook time: 20 minutes\ Servings: 4)

Ingredients:

- 1 pound frozen okra, thawed, squeeze out the water, sliced
- 1 Tablespoon flavorless oil, your choice
- 1 small white onion, sliced
- 1 garlic clove, diced
- 1 bell pepper, chopped
- 2 celery stalks, chopped
- 1 large can stewed tomatoes
- Pinch of salt and fresh ground pepper, each
- ¼ cup parmesan cheese, garnish (optional)

Directions:

1) In a large skillet, heat the oil. Sauté the onions and celery for 2 minutes. Add the garlic. Cook for 1 minute.

2) Add the okra, bell pepper, and tomatoes. Mix together.
3) Cover and cook on medium -low for 5-10 minutes, until the okra and tomatoes are fork tender.
4) Pour into a serving dish. Garnish with parmesan cheese. Serve immediately.

Nutrition Value:

- Calories: 94
- Fat: 4.7g
- Carbohydrates: 11.5g
- Protein: 3.8g

27. Roasted Garlic Cauliflower

(Prep time: 15 minutes\ Cook time: 25 minutes\ Servings: 4)

Ingredients:

- 1 large cauliflower, cut into florets
- 2 garlic cloves, minced
- 3 Tablespoons flavorless oil, your choice
- ¼ cup parmesan cheese, grated
- Pinch of salt and fresh ground pepper, each
- 1 Tablespoon fresh parsley, chopped

Directions:

1) Rinse the cauliflower, pat dry.
2) Preheat oven to 450°F.
3) Pour the oil and garlic in a large baggie.
4) Toss in the cauliflower flowers. Shake until pieces are coated.
5) Pour the mixture in a shallow baking dish. Season with salt and pepper.
6) Bake for 25 minutes, stirring after 10 minutes.

7) Pull out the baking dish, sprinkle parmesan cheese over the florets. Broil each side for 2-4 minutes, until golden brown.
8) Transfer to a serving dish. Garnish with parsley. Serve immediately.

Nutrition Value:

- Calories: 118
- Fat: 8.2g
- Carbohydrates: 8.6g
- Protein: 4.7g

28. Sesame Green Beans

(Prep time: 5 minutes\ Cook time: 25 minutes\ Servings: 4)

Ingredients:

- 1 pound fresh green beans
- 1 Tablespoon flavorless oil, your choice
- 1 Tablespoon sesame seeds
- ¼ cup chicken broth
- Pinch of salt and fresh ground pepper, each

Directions:

1) In a large skillet, heat the oil.
2) Add the sesame seeds. When they start to darken, add the green beans.
3) Pour in the broth.
4) Cover and simmer for approximately 10 minutes, until beans are slightly tender.
5) Remove the cover. Cook until the broth evaporates.
6) Pour into a serving dish. Serve immediately.

Nutrition Value:

- Calories: 333
- Fat: 31g
- Carbohydrates: 6g
- Protein: 7g

29. Gently Fried Swiss Chard

(Prep time: 15 minutes\ Cook time: 10 minutes\ Servings: 2)

Ingredients:

- Bunch of Swiss chard, stems removed, cut into bite-size pieces
- 4 slices bacon, chopped
- 2 Tablespoons butter
- 3 Tablespoons fresh squeezed lemon juice
- ½ teaspoon garlic paste
- Pinch of salt and fresh ground pepper

Directions:

1) Rinse the swiss chard, pat dry.
2) In a large skillet, add in the chopped bacon. Cook for 5 minutes,
3) Add the butter, stir until melted.
4) Add the lemon juice and garlic paste, stir until combined.
5) Toss in the Swiss chard. Stir the ingredients. Turn the heat to medium.
6) Cover and cook for 4 minutes.

7) Season with salt and pepper.
8) Pour into a serving dish. Serve immediately.

Nutrition Value:

- Calories: 56.2
- Fat: 3.7g
- Carbohydrates: 2.7g
- Protein: 39g

30. Baked Eggplant Tomato

(Prep time: 15 minutes\ Cook time: 10 minutes\ Servings: 3-4)

Ingredients:

- 1 medium sized eggplant, peeled or unpeeled, sliced into ½ inch rounds
- 2-4 Tablespoons flavorless oil, your choice
- 1 large tomato, sliced into ½ inch rounds
- Salt and fresh ground pepper
- ½ cup parmesan cheese, grated

Directions:

1) Preheat oven to 400°F.
2) Arrange the eggplant rounds on a cookie sheet in a single layer.
3) Drizzle oil lightly over eggplant slices. Season with salt and pepper.
4) Sprinkle parmesan cheese over the eggplant slices.
5) Place a slice of tomato on top of the eggplant. Drizzle oil lightly over tomato.

Season with salt and pepper. Sprinkle more parmesan cheese.
6) Bake for 10-15 minutes, until the eggplant is fork tender.
7) Serve immediately.

Nutrition Value:

- Calories: 55
- Fat: 0.3g
- Carbohydrates: 9.3g
- Protein: 3.3g

31. Mushroom Sauté

(Prep time: 5 minutes\ Cook time: 30 minutes\ Servings: 4)

Ingredients:

- 1 pound button mushrooms
- 2 Tablespoons butter
- ½ Tablespoon balsamic vinegar
- 1 garlic clove, minced
- ⅛ teaspoon dried oregano
- Salt and fresh ground pepper, each

Directions:

1) Rinse the mushrooms, pat dry. Cut off just the tip of stems.
2) In a large skillet, melt the butter. Add the garlic, balsamic vinegar, and oregano. Stir until the ingredients are combined.
3) Add the mushrooms to the skillet. Season with salt and pepper. Sauté 20 minutes, or until fork tender.
4) Serve immediately.

Nutrition Value:

- Calories: 94
- Fat: 7g
- Carbohydrates: 5.3g
- Protein: 2.3g

32. Prosciutto Wrapped Asparagus

(Prep time: 5 minutes\ Cook time: 5 minutes\ Servings: 4)

Ingredients:

- 10 asparagus spears
- 10 slices prosciutto, thinly sliced
- 1 Tablespoon flavorless oil, your choice

Directions:

1) Preheat oven to 450°F.
2) Trim off the wooden part of the asparagus. Rinse them and pat dry.
3) Starting at the bottom of the asparagus, wrap a piece of prosciutto, to the tip.
4) Drizzle olive oil over bottom of glass baking dish. Place prosciutto in single layer.
5) Bake for 5 minutes.
6) Serve immediately or at room temperature.

Nutrition Value:

- Calories: 56.2
- Fat: 3.7g
- Carbohydrates: 2.7g
- Protein: 39g

Chapter 9: Amazing Deserts

33. Chocolate Truffles

(Prep time: 10 minutes\ Cook time: 5 minutes\ Servings: 10)

Ingredients:

- 3 cups semi-sweet chocolate chips
- 14 ounce can sweetened condensed milk
- 1 Tablespoon vanilla extract
- Garnish: shredded coconut, cocoa powder, confectioner's sugar, chopped nuts

Directions:

1) In a large saucepan, heat the sweetened condensed milk.
2) Add the chocolate chips. Stir until combined.
3) Turn off the heat. Stir in vanilla extract.
4) Transfer the mixture to a glass bowl, cover with plastic wrap. (Make sure to place the plastic against the surface of the chocolate so it doesn't create a film.)
5) Chill for 3 hours.

6) Using a melon baller scooper, scoop out the chocolate.
7) Optional garnish: roll in shredded coconut, cocoa powder, confectioner's sugar or chopped nuts.
8) Chill for 30 minutes. Serve with fresh berries.

Nutrition Value:

- Calories: 53
- Fat: 2.5g
- Carbohydrates: 7.5g
- Protein: 0.9g

34. Flowerlike Rosettes

(Prep time: 15 minutes\ Cook time: 60 minutes\ Servings: 30)

Ingredients:

- 2 eggs
- 1 cup of milk
- 1 cup all-purpose flour
- 1 Tablespoon sugar
- ½ teaspoon salt
- 1 teaspoon vanilla extract
- Oil for frying: vegetable, canola, sunflower
- Garnish: Confectioner's sugar
- You will need a rosette iron

Directions:

1) In a large bowl, combine the eggs, milk and vanilla extract. Mix together.
2) In another bowl, sift the flour, sugar, and salt. Whisk together.
3) Add the wet ingredients to the dry. Stir until combined.

4) In a deep pot, pour ¼ cup of oil. Heat it up.
5) Once the oil reaches a temperature of 375°F, or very hot, dip the rosette form in the oil for 30 seconds. Drain off the excess oil from the iron. Dip the rosette into the batter, place the rosette back in the hot oil.
6) Fry the rosette until golden, approximately 30 seconds.
7) Remove the rosette from oil. Push the cooked pastry off the rosette with a fork. Place on paper towel to drain off excess oil.
8) Repeat until batter is used.
9) Once pastries are cooled, dust with confectioner's sugar.
10)   Serve with side of fresh berries.

Nutrition Value:

- Calories: 561
- Fat: 59g
- Carbohydrates: 8.2g
- Protein: 1.1g

35. Creamy Cheese Tarts
(Prep time: 40 minutes\ Cook time: 20 minutes\ Servings: 24)

Ingredients:

- 3 ounces cream cheese, room temperature
- ½ cup butter, room temperature
- 1 cup all-purpose flour
- Baking spray

Directions:

1) In a medium sized bowl, blend cream cheese until smooth.
2) Stir in the flour, continue mixing until fully blended.
3) Cover. Chill in the refrigerator for 1 hour.
4) Preheat oven to 325°F.
5) Shape the dough into 24 balls. Press them into lightly greased muffin cup tin.
6) Once your shell is ready, fill it up with whatever you like.
7) Bake for 20 minutes, until crust edges are golden brown.

8) Cool completely. Fill with fruit filling of your choice.

Nutrition Value:

- Calories: 65
- Fat: 5g
- Carbohydrates: 4g
- Protein: 1g

36. Faux Chocolate Mousse

(Prep time: 10 minutes\ Cook time: 5 minutes\ Servings: 4)

Ingredients:

- 8 ounces mascarpone cheese
- 2 Tablespoons heavy cream or whipping cream
- 1 teaspoon vanilla extract
- ¼ cup chocolate chips
- Garnish: Semi-sweet chocolate shavings

Directions:

1) Melt the chocolate chips: Either with double boiler, or in the microwave. Set aside.
2) In another bowl, mix the mascarpone cheese, vanilla extract and whipping cream until fully combined.
3) Fold the warmed chocolate into the mascarpone mixture.
4) Cover. Freeze 2 hours.
5) Serve in bowls. Garnish with whipping cream and shaved chocolate over the top.

Nutrition Value:

- Calories: 319
- Fat: 31g
- Carbohydrates: 7g
- Protein: 4g

37. Sticky Ganache

(Prep time: 5 minutes\ Cook time: 15 minutes\ Servings: 24)

Ingredients:

- 16 ounces bittersweet chocolate, chopped
- 1 cup heavy cream
- ½ cup unsalted butter

Directions:

1) In a small saucepan, heat the heavy cream.
2) Place the chopped up chocolate in a glass bowl.
3) Pour the heated cream over the chocolate.
4) Stir until the chocolate is melted and combined with the cream.
5) Add the butter. Stir until combined and shiny.
6) Cover with plastic wrap. (Make sure the cling wrap is pressed against the chocolate.)
7) Store in the refrigerator.

8) Use the Ganache whenever you need to top a dessert with something sweet.

Nutrition Value:

- Calories: 172
- Fat: 13g
- Carbohydrates: 10g
- Protein: 1.5g

38. Crunchy Pudding Cookies

(Prep time 5 minutes\ Cook time 15 minutes\ Servings:40)

Ingredients:

- 1 package Devil's Food Cake mix
- 1/3 cup vegetable oil
- 2 eggs
- ½ cup chopped walnuts
- Confectioner's sugar

Directions:

1) Preheat oven to 350°F.
2) In a medium bowl, mix the cake mix and walnuts.
3) In a measuring cup, whisk together the vegetable oil and eggs.
4) Pour the wet ingredients into the dry. Stir for 2 minutes.
5) Using a small ice cream scoop, scoop out the mix. Roll into small balls.
6) Roll the cookie dough in confectioner's sugar.
7) Place on parchment papered cookie sheet.

8) Bake for 7-9 minutes, or until edges darken.
9) Let the cookies sit for 1 minute on the cookie sheet, then transfer to a platter.
10) Cool and serve.

Nutrition Value:

- Calories: 69
- Fat: 4.2g
- Carbohydrates: 7g
- Protein: 1g

39. Fantastic Meringues
(Prep time: 20 minutes\ Cook time: 40 minutes\ Servings: 10)

Ingredients:

- 2 egg white
- ½ cup superfine sugar
- 1 teaspoon vanilla extract
- Garnish: cocoa powder

Directions:

1) Preheat oven to 300°F.
2) Line a baking sheet with parchment paper.
3) Separate the egg whites from the egg yolks. (Use the egg yolks for an omelet.)
4) In a large bowl, beat the egg whites.
5) Add the sugar.
6) Beat until egg whites form stiff peaks.
7) Add vanilla extract. Stir until combined.
8) Fill the egg white mixture in a baggie. Snip a corner of the baggie and pipe small circles onto parchment paper.
9) Bake for 35 minutes.

10)   Turn off the oven. Leave meringues in the oven until oven cools down. Meringues are ready when they are dry to the touch.
11) Option: Garnish with cocoa powder. Serve with fresh fruit compote.

Nutrition Value:

- Calories: 36
- Fat: 0g
- Carbohydrates: 8.4g
- Protein: 0.6g

40. Raw Candy

(Prep time: 20 minutes\ Cook time: 0 minutes\ Servings: 20)

Ingredients:

- 1 cup plump raisins
- 1 cup walnuts
- 1 cup pumpkin seeds
- 1 cup sunflower seeds
- 1 cup semi-sweet mini chocolate chips
- 1-2 Tablespoons honey
- Garnish: chopped almonds, shredded coconut, cocoa powder

Directions:

1) In a food processor, pulse the raisins, walnuts, pumpkin seeds, sunflower seeds, until the ingredients are broken up. (Not too long, still want chunky pieces.)
2) Pour mixture into a bowl. Add the mini chocolate chips. Stir.
3) Pour in 1 tablespoon of honey. Stir together. If the mixture seems sticky enough, don't add other tablespoon.

4) Using a small ice cream scoop, scoop out the mixture and use your hands to roll into balls. (Have a bowl of water nearby, in case your hands get too sticky.)
5) Option: roll the candy balls in chopped almonds, shredded coconut, or cocoa powder. Or leave them as they are.
6) Refrigerate for 15 minutes to firm up, or serve immediately.
7) You can refrigerate up to 3 days.

Nutrition Value:

- Calories: 45
- Fat: 3.5g
- Carbohydrates: 3.2g
- Protein: 1g

Conclusion

Once again, I would like you to thank you for downloading this book and having the patience to read it.

I do hope you had as much fun reading and experiencing the recipes as I enjoyed writing it for you.

From here on out, all you need to do is follow the rules of Low-Carb Diet, and even experiment with your very own meal plan!

Stay safe. Stay healthy and God Bless!

Lightning Source UK Ltd.
Milton Keynes UK
UKHW02f0141050118
315574UK00006B/278/P